# Longevity, Livin Living Better

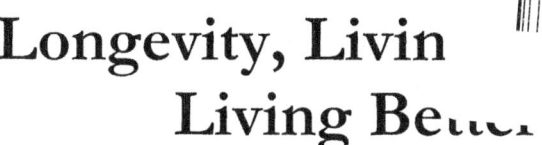

## A Practical Guide for All

Richard Trillion Mantey

Copyright © 2025

All Rights Reserved

# **Dedication**

To all those who seek to live not just longer but better—may this guide serve as a reminder that true longevity is not simply a matter of adding years to life but of adding life to your years. To the individuals who inspire change, the caregivers who give selflessly, and the dreamers who continue to hope for a healthier, brighter future. May your journey toward vitality and well-being be filled with wisdom, joy, and purpose.

To all who strive for a life of vitality, purpose, and joy, this book is for you. May it inspire you to embrace the journey toward living longer and living better—mindfully, holistically, and with intention.

And to my parents, whose unwavering love, wisdom, and guidance laid the foundation for everything I know about the importance of health, happiness, and resilience. Your example is my greatest gift. Thank you for teaching me that the true essence of life lies not just in the years we live, but in how we live them.

This book is dedicated to you with the deepest gratitude and love.

# **Acknowledgment**

I am deeply grateful to all those who have contributed to the creation of Longevity, Living Longer, Living Better: A Practical Guide for All. This book would not have been possible without the support, knowledge, and inspiration of many incredible individuals.

First, to my family—your unwavering love and encouragement have been my greatest source of strength. To my parents, thank you for teaching me the true value of health, resilience, and living with purpose.

A special thanks to the experts, health professionals, and researchers whose work paved the way for the insights shared within these pages. Your commitment to advancing the understanding of longevity has been invaluable.

To my editor and team, your dedication and belief in this project helped shape it into what it is today. Your expertise, feedback, and tireless work are deeply appreciated.

Finally, to every reader—this book is for you. May it inspire, guide, and empower you to live your longest and best life.

Thank you all for being a part of this journey.

# About the Author

Richard Trillion Mantey is a dedicated wellness advocate, researcher, and speaker with a deep passion for helping individuals live healthier, more fulfilling lives. With years of experience in the fields of nutrition, fitness, and longevity, Richard Trillion Mantey has worked with diverse populations to empower people to take control of their health and well-being at every stage of life.

Drawing on a rich background in health science and personal development, Richard Trillion Mantey integrates evidence-based practices with practical, real-world solutions to support sustainable wellness. As an expert in the aging process, Richard Trillion Mantey focuses on the intersection of physical, mental, and emotional health, emphasizing a holistic approach to longevity that encourages balanced living and mindful aging.

Having authored several articles, conducted workshops, and collaborated with wellness organizations, Richard Trillion Mantey has earned a reputation for delivering insightful, easy-to-understand advice that resonates with readers of all ages. Longevity, Living Longer, Living Better is the culmination of Richard Trillion Mantey's years of study and work in the wellness field, providing readers with the tools they need to not only add years to their lives but also enhance the quality of those years.

With a commitment to promoting lifelong health and happiness, Richard Trillion Mantey continues to inspire and educate individuals around the world on how to live their best, most vibrant lives.

# Book Description

**Longevity, Living Longer, Living Better: A Practical Guide for All**

Unlock the secrets to a healthier, more vibrant life with Longevity, Living Longer, Living Better. This practical guide offers science-backed insights, actionable tips, and lifestyle strategies designed to help you optimize your well-being and enjoy a longer, more fulfilling life—no matter your age or stage in life.

Whether you're seeking to boost your energy, improve your mental clarity, or simply live a more balanced life, this book provides easy-to-follow advice rooted in the latest research on aging, nutrition, exercise, and emotional health.

Inside, you'll discover:

- Simple yet effective habits to support long-term health and vitality.
- The importance of nutrition and exercise for maintaining a strong, active body.
- Mindset shifts that promote resilience, happiness, and mental well-being.
- Practical strategies for reducing stress, improving sleep, and fostering social connections.
- How to cultivate a lifestyle that embraces aging gracefully while maximizing your quality of life.

Written for readers of all ages, Longevity, Living Longer, Living Better offers a holistic approach to aging and wellness. Embrace the journey of living not just longer but better—empowered with the knowledge to make healthier choices and live your best life every day.

Take control of your future today and start living with greater purpose and joy!

# Contents

Dedication ................................................................................. i

Acknowledgment ..................................................................... ii

About the Author .................................................................... iii

Book Description ..................................................................... v

Chapter 1: Understanding Longevity ..................................... 1

Chapter 2: Nutrition for a Longer Life ................................. 20

Chapter 3: Physical Activity and Longevity ........................ 26

Chapter 4: Mental Well-being and Longevity ..................... 32

Chapter 5: Social Connections and Longevity .................... 41

Chapter 6: Sleep and Recovery ............................................. 47

Chapter 7: Preventive Healthcare ......................................... 53

Chapter 8: Healthy Habits for Everyday Life ...................... 57

Chapter 9: Embracing Change and Adaptability ................ 63

Chapter 10: Inspiring Stories of Longevity ......................... 69

Chapter 11: Creating Your Personal Longevity Plan ......... 75

Chapter 12: : Conclusion: A Holistic Approach to Living Longer, Living Better ............................................................. 81

# Chapter 1
## Understanding Longevity

**The Science of Aging**

Aging is a complex biological process that has intrigued scientists and philosophers for centuries. At its core, aging can be understood as the gradual decline of physiological functions and the increased vulnerability to diseases. This process is influenced by a myriad of factors, including genetics, environmental conditions, lifestyle choices, and even social interactions. Researchers have identified several theories of aging, such as the free radical theory, which suggests that oxidative damage from free radicals contributes to cellular aging, and the telomere shortening theory, which posits that the protective caps on chromosomes shorten with each cell division, eventually leading to cell senescence.

One of the key components of the aging process is the role of cellular senescence. As cells divide, they can become senescent due to various stressors, including DNA damage and telomere shortening. Senescent cells no longer divide and can secrete pro-inflammatory factors contributing to tissue dysfunction and age-related diseases. This accumulation of senescent cells is thought to play a significant role in the development of age-related conditions such as cancer, cardiovascular disease, and neurodegenerative disorders.

Understanding the mechanisms behind cellular senescence is crucial in developing potential therapies aimed at rejuvenating aging tissues and improving overall health.

Another important aspect of the science of aging is the impact of lifestyle factors on longevity. Research has shown that diet, physical activity, and stress management significantly influence the aging process. For instance, diets rich in antioxidants, such as fruits and vegetables, can help mitigate oxidative stress, while regular physical activity promotes cardiovascular health and maintains muscle mass. Moreover, mindfulness practices and social connections have been linked to reduced stress levels and improved emotional well-being, further enhancing the quality of life as one ages. This evidence underscores the importance of adopting healthy habits to support longevity and overall health.

The field of gerontology continues to advance with ongoing research aimed at understanding the biological mechanisms of aging. Recent breakthroughs in biotechnology and genetics have opened new avenues for potential interventions. For example, studies involving caloric restriction have shown promising results in extending lifespan in various organisms by slowing down metabolic processes and enhancing cellular repair mechanisms. Additionally, advancements in gene therapy and regenerative medicine offer hope for reversing some aspects of aging, potentially allowing individuals to maintain vitality and health well into their later years.

Ultimately, the science of aging is not just about adding years to life but enhancing the quality of those years. As our understanding of the aging process deepens, it becomes increasingly clear that a multifaceted approach—incorporating biological, psychological, and social elements—will be essential in promoting longevity and well-being. By embracing this knowledge and implementing practical strategies, individuals can take proactive steps toward living longer, healthier lives, making the most of their golden years while enjoying the journey along the way.

## Historical Perspectives on Longevity

The quest for longevity has captivated human beings throughout history, influencing cultures, philosophies, and scientific endeavors. Ancient civilizations often attributed longevity to divine favor or the pursuit of knowledge. For instance, the Chinese philosopher Laozi emphasized harmony with nature and a balanced lifestyle as keys to a long life. Similarly, the Greeks celebrated the pursuit of virtue and wisdom, often linking these ideals to a greater lifespan. This historical perspective highlights how societies have long recognized the interplay between lifestyle, health, and longevity.

In the Middle Ages, the understanding of longevity began to shift as religious and superstitious beliefs intertwined with medical knowledge. Many people viewed longevity as a reward for piety or moral living. The writings of figures such as Hildegard of Bingen showcased herbal remedies and holistic approaches to health, suggesting that a natural diet and spiritual well-being could extend life. Yet, this era also faced challenges such as plagues and poor hygiene, which often counteracted efforts to live longer. Historical records from this period illustrate the tension between emerging medical practices and the prevailing belief systems.

The Enlightenment marked a significant turning point in the study of longevity, as empirical observation and scientific inquiry began to gain prominence. Scholars like Thomas Sydenham and Giovanni Maria Lancisi started to document the effects of diet, exercise, and environment on health. This period also saw the birth of modern medicine, with advancements in understanding anatomy and disease. The increased focus on human anatomy and physiology laid the groundwork for future research into the biological aspects of aging, emphasizing that longevity was not merely a matter of fate but could be influenced by lifestyle choices.

The 20th century brought a surge of interest in longevity, particularly with the advent of modern medicine and public health initiatives. Vaccinations, improved sanitation, and advancements in nutrition contributed to dramatic increases in life expectancy. Researchers began to explore the genetic factors that might influence aging, leading to the discovery of longevity genes. The study of centenarians and their lifestyles further fueled interest in the habits that contribute to longer, healthier lives. This era highlighted the importance of medical advancements and personal choices in achieving longevity.

Today, the pursuit of longevity remains a central theme in health discussions, influenced by historical perspectives and modern research. As we embrace advancements in genetics, biotechnology, and lifestyle medicine, we also draw from the lessons of the past. The integration of traditional knowledge with contemporary science emphasizes a holistic approach to health and longevity. Understanding historical perspectives on longevity not only enriches our appreciation for the complexities of aging but also empowers us to make informed choices as we strive for longer, healthier lives.

## Myths and Misconceptions

Myths and misconceptions surrounding longevity often cloud our understanding of what it truly means to live a long and healthy life. Many people believe that longevity is solely a matter of genetics, assuming that those who have long-lived relatives are automatically destined for the same fate. While genetics do play a role in determining lifespan, environmental factors, lifestyle choices, and social connections are equally, if not more, significant. Research shows that adopting healthy habits such as a balanced diet, regular physical activity, and maintaining strong social ties can have a profound impact on one's longevity, regardless of genetic predisposition.

Another common myth is that aging inevitably leads to declining health and vitality. This notion can discourage individuals from taking proactive steps toward healthy living as they age. In reality, many people remain active and healthy well into their later years. The concept of "successful aging" emphasizes the importance of maintaining physical, mental, and emotional well-being as one grows older. Engaging in regular exercise, pursuing hobbies, and fostering relationships can enhance the quality of life and counteract many age-related health issues, challenging the stereotype of aging as a period of decline.

Moreover, there is a widespread belief that specific diets or supplements can guarantee longevity. While proper nutrition is essential for maintaining health, no magical food or pill can extend life indefinitely. The key lies in a well-rounded diet rich in fruits, vegetables, whole grains, and lean proteins. The Mediterranean diet has also gained attention for its potential health benefits, but it is not a one-size-fits-all solution. Individual dietary needs can vary greatly, and it is crucial to approach nutrition with a personalized perspective rather than relying on trending diets or quick fixes.

Another misconception is that longevity is primarily about avoiding risk factors, such as smoking or excessive alcohol consumption. While reducing these risks is vital, focusing on positive lifestyle choices that promote health is equally important. Engaging in regular physical activity, nurturing social connections, and practicing stress management techniques contribute significantly to overall well-being. The emphasis should be on creating a balanced lifestyle that includes preventive measures alongside proactive health-enhancing habits rather than solely avoiding negatives.

Finally, many people believe that achieving longevity requires extreme measures, such as rigorous exercise regimens or strict dietary restrictions. In contrast, sustainable changes that incorporate moderate exercise and balanced eating can lead to better long-term outcomes. Finding enjoyable physical activities and making gradual dietary adjustments can foster a sense of well-being and prevent burnout. The journey towards a longer, healthier life should be viewed as an attainable and enjoyable process rather than a daunting challenge. By dispelling these myths and misconceptions, individuals can better understand and embrace strategies that contribute to a fulfilling and extended life.

## The Subconscious Mind

Imagine living to be over a hundred years old, in good health, with a mind as sharp as a tack. It's not merely a dream; it's a potential reality. You may assume this is a plot from a sci-fi novel, but it isn't. It's the reality that our minds, both conscious and subconscious, play a crucial role in our longevity and our capacity to live long, energetic lives. And today, we will investigate the secret of longevity, and the profound impact our minds have over it. Longevity isn't just about the number of candles on your birthday cake. It's about the quality of those years. It's about maintaining our physical health, indeed, but also our mental sharpness, our emotional equilibrium, and our sense of purpose. With all its intricacy, the human mind is at the heart of it all.

Here's a surprising fact: Did you know you can program your subconscious mind through repetition to influence your lifespan? We're not just talking about genetics or the ideal diet here. Your mind, thoughts, and beliefs all play a part. An expanding body of research suggests that positive mental attitudes can augment the immune system, decrease the risk of chronic diseases, and even decelerate the aging process.

Yes, the secret of longevity might not lie in a magic pill but in the power of the mind. It's about harnessing the potential of our conscious and subconscious thoughts to shape our reality, influence our physical health, and, ultimately, extend our lives.

But how does this work? How can our mind, something so intangible, have such a tangible effect on our lifespan? It's a fascinating journey that we're about to undertake, exploring the power of the conscious mind, the influence of the subconscious mind, and the practical steps we can take to tap into this potential for longevity, including the programming of our subconscious mind through repetition.

By understanding how our mind works, we can tap into its power to live longer, healthier lives. And that's not just an optimistic statement. It's a fact supported by science. The secret of longevity resides within us, in the power of our minds. Let's uncover it together. The Conscious Mind; "Let's delve into the conscious mind, the part of our mind that we're most familiar with." The conscious mind is like the captain of a ship. It's where we make decisions, solve problems, and control our physical actions. But what exactly is it?

Picture an iceberg. The tip of the iceberg that's visible above the water represents our conscious mind, while the vast majority underneath represents our subconscious mind. Our conscious mind is what we are aware of at any given moment, our thoughts, feelings, and actions, and we can actively influence and direct them with our will. The conscious mind is a fascinating part of our cognition. It's the part of our mind responsible for logic and reasoning. If you're deciding whether or not to have that piece of cake, trying to figure out the quickest route to work, or even deciding whether you should lift your hand to reach for a n, your conscious mind is at work. Our conscious mind also plays a significant role in our emotions, thoughts, and memories. It's the part of our mind that acknowledges emotions, allows thoughts to be articulated into words, and recalls memories from the past. This is why you can remember your first day at school, feel happy when you see a loved one, or articulate your thoughts into a coherent sentence.

But it's not just about thoughts and emotions. Our conscious mind also controls our physical actions. When you decide to walk, talk, run, or jump, your conscious mind is in control. It's like the director of a movie, coordinating the actions and reactions of our body in response to our thoughts and perceptions. However, the conscious mind has its limitations. It can only process a limited amount of information at a time.

Imagine trying to solve a complex mathematical equation while also trying to remember a list of twenty items and deciding what to have for dinner. It's simply too much for the conscious mind to handle at once. And here's where it gets interesting. While our conscious mind is a powerful tool, it's not the only player in the game. Our subconscious mind, which is the larger part of the iceberg submerged under the water, holds a significant amount of untapped power that we can harness to influence our health, well-being, and even longevity. Our conscious mind plays a crucial role in our daily lives. But it's not the only player in the game of longevity.

## Programming Your Subconscious Mind for Longevity

Did you know you can program your subconscious mind to live up to 200 years? That's right, the subconscious mind, the hidden powerhouse of our cognition, is highly influential and can be programmed to promote longevity. The subconscious mind is like soft clay, ready to be molded by our thoughts, beliefs, and experiences. It operates under the radar, silently influencing our decisions, actions, and reactions.

But here's the exciting part - we can influence it. We can program our subconscious mind to foster positive beliefs and habits that enhance our health and longevity. So, how do we do that? We can use several techniques to program our subconscious mind for longevity. These include affirmations, visualization, and meditation. Affirmations are positive statements that we repeat to ourselves to instill positive beliefs and attitudes. For example, saying, "I am healthy and full of vitality," can help instill a belief in our subconscious mind that we are indeed healthy and full of life. Visualization involves creating a mental image of a desired outcome.

For instance, visualizing ourselves as lively, active, and healthy even in old age can help program our subconscious mind to strive towards this vision. Conversely, meditation helps us tap into our subconscious mind and influence its programming directly. Regular meditation can cultivate a sense of inner peace, reduce stress, and promote overall well-being, all of which can contribute to longevity. The potential of the subconscious mind to extend our lifespan is immense. It's like a hidden treasure chest waiting to be unlocked.

Our subconscious mind stores our past experiences and memories and holds the key to our future. By programming our subconscious mind for longevity, we can influence our beliefs, actions, and habits to promote health and longevity. It's like planting a seed in fertile soil. With the right care and nourishment, this seed can grow into a strong, healthy tree capable of withstanding the test of time. "With the right programming, our subconscious mind can be a powerful tool for longevity."

Just like a computer, our mind can be programmed to achieve specific outcomes. When it comes to longevity, the subconscious mind is a vital player. By harnessing its power, we can unlock the secrets to a long, healthy, and fulfilling life. So why not start today? After all, the key to longevity lies not just in our genes but also in our minds.

**The Subconscious Mind**

Now, let's explore the mysterious world of the subconscious mind. The subconscious mind is like the backstage crew of a theater production, constantly working behind the scenes to ensure everything runs smoothly. Though not as visible as the conscious mind, it plays a critical role in shaping our lives, our health, and, ultimately, our longevity.

So, what exactly is the subconscious mind? It is a part of our mind that is not in focal awareness. It's an automatic, hidden force that shapes how we perceive our reality. It's a storage room for our past experiences, deepest desires, and most profound fears. The scriptwriter pens the narrative of our lives based on the beliefs and experiences we've accumulated over time.

One of the primary functions of the subconscious mind is memory storage. Every moment we've ever experienced and every emotion we've ever felt is stored in the vast library of our subconscious mind. This library constantly influences our decisions, actions, and reactions in ways we may not even be aware of. The subconscious mind is also the home of our habits. It's where the patterns of our behavior are formed and solidified.

Ever wondered why you automatically reach for a toothbrush first thing in the morning or why you instinctively know how to ride a bike, even if you haven't done it for years? That's your subconscious mind at work, taking over tasks that have become routine so your conscious mind can focus on other things.

Our personality traits, too, are deeply ingrained in our subconscious. Our tendencies, our reactions, and our preferences are all influenced by this powerful force. It's why we are drawn to certain people, react in certain ways to certain situations, and have the preferences we do. The subconscious mind also regulates our bodily functions. The silent conductor keeps the orchestra of our bodily systems in harmony. It regulates our heart rate, our breathing, and our digestion - all without our conscious control. The subconscious mind keeps our bodies functioning optimally, allowing us to live, grow, and thrive.

What's fascinating is that the subconscious mind can also be influenced. Through practices like meditation, affirmations, and visualization, we can program our subconscious mind to foster positive beliefs and habits that can enhance our health and longevity. In essence, the subconscious mind is our silent partner in the journey of life. It's the force that keeps our bodies running smoothly, shapes our personalities, forms our habits, and stores our memories. It's constantly influencing our decisions, actions, and reactions, shaping our lives' trajectory.

"Our subconscious mind might be less apparent, but its influence on our longevity is just as significant as our conscious mind's." Understanding and harnessing the power of our subconscious mind can unlock the secrets to a long, healthy, and fulfilling life. The Power of the Mind for Longevity; "So, how do these two parts of the mind contribute to our longevity?" Let's delve into this fascinating topic.

Both the conscious and subconscious mind play significant roles in determining our longevity. They are like two sides of the same coin, each with its unique influence on our health and life span. Starting with the conscious mind is the part of our mind that deals with our active thought processes. It's here that we make decisions, form opinions, and engage in problem-solving. It's our conscious mind that decides to choose a salad over a burger or to take the stairs instead of the elevator. These decisions, as minor as they may seem, collectively contribute to our overall health and longevity.

Stress, as we know, has a direct impact on our health. It can lead to a host of physical and mental ailments, from heart disease to depression. By consciously choosing to manage our stress levels, perhaps through techniques like meditation, exercise, or simply taking a break when we need it, we can mitigate the harmful effects of stress on our health and extend our lifespan.

Now, let's turn our attention to the subconscious mind. This is the part of our mind that operates below our level of conscious awareness. The subconscious mind is incredibly powerful and can significantly influence our longevity. It's like the autopilot of our mind, guiding our actions and behaviors without us even realizing it. Our eating habits, our exercise routines, and even our thought patterns are all largely driven by our subconscious mind.

So, how can we leverage this to promote longevity? The key lies in positive thinking and forming healthy habits. When we cultivate positive thought patterns, they seep into our subconscious, influencing our attitudes and behaviors in beneficial ways. For instance, a positive outlook can motivate us to take better care of our health, to be more physically active, and to eat a balanced diet. Similarly, when we form healthy habits, they become ingrained in our subconscious mind.

Over time, these habits become second nature to us, requiring little to no conscious effort. This could be anything from daily exercise to getting enough sleep to drinking plenty of water. The subconscious mind is also instrumental in managing stress. When we adopt stress management techniques like meditation or deep breathing, over time, these practices become automatic responses to stress, greatly reducing its detrimental effects on our health. In essence, our mind, both conscious and subconscious, holds immense power over our health and longevity.

By harnessing this power, by consciously making healthier choices and cultivating positive, health-promoting habits that seep into our subconscious, we can significantly enhance our longevity. "Harnessing the power of our mind is key to unlocking a longer, healthier life."

## Programming the Subconscious for Longevity

Moving onward, (let us scrutinize a significant notion: programming the subconscious mind for longevity and even deciding our lifespan.) The subconscious mind is indeed akin to a fertile garden; the seeds we embed within it will gently nurture and expand. By seeds of positivity, health, and longevity, our subconscious mind will work unceasingly to bring these into existence in our lives.

A highly effective method to our subconscious mind is through repetition. This is attributable to our subconscious mind's capacity to learn through patterns and repeated occurrences. The continual repetition of a thought, action, or behavior in our subconscious mind is done through repetition. This is attributable to our subconscious mind's capacity to learn to cultivate a habit of exercising daily. Start setting a precise, attainable goal.

For instance, you could aim to exercise for 20 minutes each day. Initially, it would require conscious effort and determination to stick to this routine. However, as you execute this action over time, it will seep into your subconscious mind, and daily exercise will eventually become a natural, effortless activity. Likewise, we can use repetition to nurture positive thinking patterns. By consistently fostering positive thoughts about our health and longevity, we can harmonize our subconscious mind with these thoughts. Intriguingly, our subconscious mind does not differentiate between reality and imagination.

Therefore, if we consistently visualize ourselves as healthy, vibrant, and living a long life, our subconscious mind will endeavor to make these images a reality. To facilitate this process, we can use positive affirmations, empowering statements we repeat daily. Affirmations such as "I am healthy and full of vitality" or "Every day, in every way, I am getting healthier and healthier," I am blessed with a vibrant, long life full of vitality and health. Every cell in my body is healthy, strong, and regenerating with each passing day.

I am deeply connected to the universal energy that supports my longevity and wellness.

My body is in perfect harmony, and I am continually growing stronger, healthier, and more youthful.

I honor my body, mind, and spirit, nourishing them for a long, fulfilling life.

I attract abundance in all forms, including the gift of a long and prosperous life.

I radiate energy, youthfulness, and vitality every day, and my life grows longer with each breath.

Every decision I make supports my health, longevity, and well-being.

I am grateful for the many years of vibrant life ahead of me.

My lifespan is extended with every moment of joy, peace, and gratitude I experience. This can significantly impact our subconscious mind, influencing our attitudes, behaviors, and, ultimately, our health and longevity. In addition, by regularly asserting statements like "I will live a long and healthy life," we can program our subconscious mind to determine our lifespan. But there's more to it. The subconscious mind can be further programmed by visualizing by visualizing our desired lifespan repeatedly. Imagine yourself living and thriving to a ripe old age, enjoying the richness of life. This consistent focus on a long, healthy life will eventually become a deep-seated belief in your subconscious mind, influencing not only your lifestyle choices but also your physical health. Using repetition to program our subconscious mind is a mighty instrument in our quest for longevity and lifespan regulation."

## Practical Tips for Longevity

"Now that we understand the role of our mind in longevity, what steps can we take to use this knowledge?" Our first practical tip is to maintain a positive mindset. Our thoughts shape our reality, and we can influence our physical health by consciously choosing to think positively. Positive thinking can boost our immunity, reduce stress, and even slow the aging process. To cultivate a positive mindset, try to modify your thought patterns. For instance, instead of thinking, "I always get sick," reframe it to, "I am building a stronger immune system."

Next, let's talk about managing stress. Chronic stress can wreak havoc on our bodies, accelerating the aging process and increasing the risk of disease. It's essential to find effective ways to manage stress for a longer, healthier life. Simple techniques like deep breathing, meditation, and yoga can help us relax and keep stress at bay. Moreover, engaging in hobbies that bring joy and fulfillment can also act as a stress buster.

Remember, it's not about eliminating stress; how we manage it matters. Thirdly, let's discuss the importance of cultivating healthy habits. The conscious mind can help us make better choices when it comes to our diet, exercise, and sleep. Eating a balanced diet rich in fruits, vegetables, whole grains, and lean proteins can provide our bodies with the nutrients needed for optimal health and longevity.

Regular exercise, on the other hand, can keep our bodies fit and our minds sharp. Aim for at least thirty minutes of physical activity each day. And don't forget about sleep. Quality sleep is crucial for our bodies to restore and rejuvenate. Try to get seven to nine hours of sleep each night. Another tip is to practice mindfulness. Mindfulness is about staying present and fully engaged in the moment. It allows us to be more aware of our thoughts and feelings without getting caught up in them. This awareness can help us better manage our emotions and reduce stress, contributing to longevity.

Last but not least, the power of visualization shouldn't be underestimated. Our subconscious mind responds powerfully to images, so visualizing ourselves as healthy and vibrant can have a positive impact on our physical health. Spend a few minutes each day imagining yourself living a long, healthy life.

In conclusion, longevity isn't just about genetics or luck. It's about harnessing the power of our conscious and subconscious minds to influence our physical health. By maintaining a positive mindset, managing stress, cultivating healthy habits, practicing mindfulness, and using visualization, we can tap into this power to increase our lifespan. "With these tips, we can tap into the power of our mind to increase our lifespan."

# Chapter 2
# Nutrition for a Longer Life

**Essential Nutrients and Their Roles**

Essential nutrients are the building blocks of a healthy diet and play a pivotal role in maintaining overall health and longevity. These nutrients are categorized into macronutrients and micronutrients. Macronutrients include carbohydrates, proteins, and fats, which provide energy and support bodily functions. Micronutrients, comprising vitamins and minerals, are crucial for various biochemical processes. Understanding the roles these nutrients play can empower individuals to make informed dietary choices that promote longevity.

Carbohydrates are often misunderstood, but they are essential for providing energy to the body. They are classified into simple and complex carbohydrates, with complex carbohydrates being the preferred source because they provide sustained energy and are rich in fiber. Fiber not only aids digestion but also helps regulate blood sugar levels and lowers cholesterol. A diet rich in whole grains, fruits, and vegetables ensures an adequate intake of carbohydrates, which supports both physical activity and cognitive function, contributing to a longer and healthier life.

Proteins are vital for the repair and growth of tissues. They are made up of essential amino acids, some of which must be obtained through diet. Adequate protein intake is linked to muscle maintenance, immune function, and hormone production. High-quality protein sources include lean meats, fish, dairy, legumes, and nuts. Incorporating a variety of protein sources into meals can help ensure that the body receives all essential amino acids, supporting overall health and longevity.

Fats are often demonized in modern diets, yet they are a crucial component of a balanced nutrition strategy. Healthy fats, such as those found in avocados, nuts, seeds, and olive oil, play a significant role in brain health, hormone regulation, and nutrient absorption. Omega-3 fatty acids, in particular, are known for their anti-inflammatory properties and have been linked to a reduced risk of chronic diseases. Including healthy fats in the diet can enhance overall well-being and support a longer lifespan.

Micronutrients, which include vitamins and minerals, are equally important for health. Vitamins such as A, C, D, E, and the B-complex group support a range of bodily functions, from immune response to energy metabolism. Minerals like calcium, potassium, and magnesium are critical for bone health, muscle function, and maintaining fluid balance. A diet rich in colorful fruits and vegetables, whole grains, and lean proteins can help ensure an adequate intake of these essential micronutrients. By understanding the diverse roles of these essential nutrients, individuals can make dietary choices that enhance their quality of life and promote longevity.

## The Mediterranean Diet

The Mediterranean diet is often heralded as one of the world's healthiest dietary patterns, contributing to improved health and longevity. Originating from the traditional eating practices of countries bordering the Mediterranean Sea, this diet emphasizes fresh, seasonal, and local foods. It primarily consists of fruits, vegetables, whole grains, legumes, nuts, and healthy fats, particularly olive oil. Fish and seafood are consumed regularly, while red meats and processed foods are limited. This balance of nutrients plays a crucial role in supporting overall health and well-being.

One of the key components of the Mediterranean diet is its focus on healthy fats, specifically monounsaturated fats found in olive oil. These fats are known to promote heart health by reducing bad cholesterol levels and lowering the risk of cardiovascular diseases. Additionally, the diet includes omega-3 fatty acids from fish, which have been linked to improved brain health and reduced inflammation. Incorporating these fats into daily meals enhances flavor and provides essential nutrients that contribute to longevity.

Fruits and vegetables, which form the foundation of the Mediterranean diet, are packed with vitamins, minerals, and antioxidants. These nutrient-dense foods help combat oxidative stress and inflammation, which are associated with aging and chronic diseases. A diverse range of colorful produce ensures that individuals receive a broad spectrum of beneficial compounds. Regular consumption of plant-based foods has been linked to reduced risks of conditions such as heart disease, diabetes, and certain types of cancer, further supporting the premise of living a longer and healthier life.

In addition to the nutritional aspects, the Mediterranean diet emphasizes the importance of social eating and physical activity. Meals are often enjoyed with family and friends, fostering a sense of community and psychological well-being. This social interaction can reduce stress and promote healthier eating habits. Furthermore, the Mediterranean lifestyle encourages regular physical activity, whether through walking, gardening, or other forms of exercise. These factors combined contribute to a holistic approach to health, reinforcing the connection between diet, lifestyle, and longevity.

Adopting the Mediterranean diet does not require drastic changes; rather, it encourages gradual shifts toward healthier choices. Simple steps to embrace this way of eating include replacing butter with olive oil, incorporating more plant-based meals into the week, and choosing fish over red meat. Individuals can significantly enhance their health and increase their chances of living longer by focusing on whole, minimally processed foods and enjoying meals in a communal setting. This diet serves as a practical guide for anyone seeking to improve their overall well-being while enjoying the pleasures of flavorful and nourishing meals.

**Plant-Based Eating**

Plant-based eating has gained significant attention in recent years, not only for its environmental benefits but also for its potential to promote longevity and overall well-being. This dietary approach emphasizes the consumption of whole, minimally processed plant foods, including fruits, vegetables, whole grains, legumes, nuts, and seeds. By prioritizing these foods, individuals can nourish their bodies with essential nutrients while reducing the intake of harmful substances often found in animal products, such as saturated fats and cholesterol.

Numerous studies have linked plant-based diets to a reduced risk of chronic diseases, such as heart disease, diabetes, and certain cancers. These conditions are prevalent in many populations and can significantly impact longevity. The high fiber content of plant foods promotes healthy digestion and can help maintain a healthy weight, both of which are crucial for preventing chronic illnesses. Additionally, many plant foods are rich in antioxidants and phytonutrients, which help combat oxidative stress and inflammation in the body, two key factors that contribute to aging and disease.

Transitioning to a plant-based diet doesn't have to be an all-or-nothing approach. Individuals can start by incorporating more plant-based meals into their weekly routines. Simple changes, such as replacing meat with legumes in recipes or introducing a variety of vegetables to daily meals, can make a significant difference. Exploring new plant-based recipes can also make the process enjoyable and satisfying. Many people find that as they experiment with different flavors and textures, they begin to appreciate the diversity and richness of plant-based eating.

In addition to its health benefits, plant-based eating can also be a sustainable choice for the planet. The production of plant foods generally requires fewer resources and generates lower greenhouse gas emissions compared to animal agriculture. By choosing more plant-based options, individuals are investing in their health and contributing to a more sustainable food system. This connection between personal health and environmental impact resonates with a growing number of people, particularly those interested in living longer, healthier lives.

Ultimately, embracing a plant-based diet can be a powerful strategy for enhancing longevity and improving quality of life. By focusing on nutrient-dense, whole foods, individuals can support their bodies in the quest for optimal health. As more research continues to emerge on the benefits of plant-based eating, it becomes increasingly clear that this dietary choice is not just a trend but a viable path toward a longer, healthier future.

# Chapter 3
# Physical Activity and Longevity

**Importance of Regular Exercise**

Regular exercise plays a crucial role in maintaining overall health and well-being, making it a fundamental component of a long and fulfilling life. Engaging in physical activity helps to manage weight, reduce the risk of chronic diseases, and improve mental health. Studies have shown that individuals who incorporate regular exercise into their routines experience lower rates of conditions such as heart disease, diabetes, and certain cancers. This preventative approach enhances quality of life and contributes to longevity, highlighting the necessity of making exercise a priority.

One of the most significant benefits of regular exercise is its impact on cardiovascular health. Engaging in aerobic activities, such as walking, running, or cycling, strengthens the heart, improves circulation, and lowers blood pressure. A healthy heart is essential for maintaining adequate blood flow and oxygen delivery throughout the body. By reducing the risk of heart disease, stroke, and other cardiovascular issues, exercise becomes an indispensable tool in promoting a longer life. Furthermore, maintaining a healthy heart can enhance energy levels and overall vitality, making it easier to engage in daily activities.

In addition to physical benefits, regular exercise has profound effects on mental health. Physical activity stimulates the release of endorphins, often referred to as "feel-good" hormones, which can alleviate symptoms of anxiety and depression. Exercise also fosters improved cognitive function and memory retention, reducing the likelihood of age-related cognitive decline. As people age, maintaining mental sharpness becomes increasingly important, and regular exercise serves as a powerful ally in achieving this goal. By promoting mental clarity and emotional resilience, exercise contributes to a holistic approach to longevity.

Social interaction is another vital aspect of regular exercise that can enhance life satisfaction and longevity. Participating in group activities, such as fitness classes or team sports, fosters connections with others, creating a sense of community and belonging. These social bonds can lead to increased motivation to stay active, as well as emotional support that enhances overall well-being. Engaging in exercise with friends or family makes physical activity more enjoyable and reinforces positive habits that contribute to a longer, healthier life.

Lastly, establishing a regular exercise routine instills discipline and a sense of accomplishment. Whether related to strength, endurance, or flexibility, setting and achieving fitness goals can boost self-esteem and provide a sense of purpose. This positive reinforcement encourages individuals to continue prioritizing their health, leading to sustained physical activity over the long term. By recognizing the importance of regular exercise, individuals can take proactive steps towards a healthier lifestyle, significantly impacting their longevity and overall quality of life.

## Types of Exercises for All Ages

Exercise is a fundamental component of a healthy lifestyle, contributing significantly to longevity and overall well-being. Understanding the various types of exercises available can help individuals of all ages find activities that suit their interests and physical capabilities. From childhood through later adulthood, engaging in appropriate forms of exercise can foster physical fitness, mental health, and social interaction, all of which are vital for living a longer, healthier life.

Physical activity is essential for the growth, development, and establishment of lifelong healthy habits for children and adolescents. Aerobic exercises, such as running, swimming, and cycling, promote cardiovascular health, while strength training activities, like bodyweight exercises or resistance bands, can aid in building muscle and improving bone density. Moreover, activities that enhance flexibility and coordination, such as dance, gymnastics, or martial arts, can contribute to overall fitness and body awareness. Regular participation in sports or group activities supports physical health and fosters teamwork and social skills.

As individuals transition into adulthood, the focus of exercise may shift to maintaining fitness levels, managing stress, and preventing chronic diseases. A balanced exercise regimen that includes aerobic exercises, strength training, and flexibility routines is ideal. Activities like jogging, brisk walking, and group fitness classes can enhance cardiovascular fitness and endurance, while weightlifting or resistance training helps preserve muscle mass and metabolic health. Moreover, integrating yoga or Pilates into a weekly routine can improve flexibility, balance, and mental clarity, which are essential for navigating the complexities of adult life.

For older adults, exercise remains crucial for maintaining independence and quality of life. Low-impact aerobic exercises, such as walking, swimming, or cycling, can be beneficial for heart health without placing excessive strain on joints. Strength training with light weights or resistance bands helps combat muscle loss associated with aging, while balance exercises, such as tai chi or specific stability routines, can reduce the risk of falls. Additionally, engaging in social exercise activities, such as group classes or walking clubs, can enhance motivation and provide essential social interaction, which is vital for emotional well-being.

In conclusion, exercise can and should be adapted to suit the needs and abilities of individuals at different life stages. From playful activities for children to balanced routines for adults and gentle exercises for seniors, there is an array of options available. The key is to find enjoyable activities that promote consistency and encourage a lifelong commitment to physical fitness. By embracing the diverse types of exercises available, individuals can significantly enhance their quality of life and increase their chances of living longer, healthier lives.

## Incorporating Movement into Daily Life

Incorporating movement into daily life is essential for enhancing overall well-being and longevity. Regular physical activity contributes to improved cardiovascular health, stronger muscles, and better joint function. However, many people struggle to find time for formal exercise routines. The good news is that movement can be integrated seamlessly into everyday activities. By making small adjustments to daily habits, individuals can significantly increase their physical activity levels without needing a structured workout.

One effective way to incorporate movement is through active commuting. For those who live within a reasonable distance from work or school, walking or cycling instead of driving can add valuable exercise to the day. Public transportation users can also benefit by getting off a stop early and walking the remaining distance. This approach enhances physical fitness, reduces stress, and promotes a sense of community by engaging with the environment and fellow commuters.

Another opportunity for movement lies in household chores. Activities such as vacuuming, gardening, and washing windows can all be turned into mini-workouts. Instead of viewing these tasks as mundane obligations, individuals can embrace them as a chance to stay active. For example, gardening provides a full-body workout, improving strength and flexibility while allowing individuals to connect with nature. Moreover, cleaning can be approached with a more vigorous technique, turning it into a calorie-burning session.

Incorporating movement into social interactions is another effective strategy. Consider organizing walking meetups or group fitness classes instead of meeting friends for coffee or a meal. This not only enhances social bonds but also makes the experience more enjoyable. Engaging in activities like dancing, hiking, or playing sports fosters a sense of camaraderie while keeping everyone physically active. These social movements can create lasting memories and motivate individuals to maintain an active lifestyle.

Lastly, technology can play a significant role in promoting movement. Wearable fitness trackers and smartphone apps can help individuals monitor their activity levels and set achievable movement goals. Many of these tools offer reminders to stand up, stretch, or take short walks throughout the day. By leveraging technology, people can stay accountable and motivated to incorporate more movement into their routines. This proactive approach to daily activity can lead to a healthier, happier life, ultimately contributing to a longer and more fulfilling existence.

# Chapter 4
# Mental Well-being and Longevity

**The Mind-Body Connection**

The mind-body connection refers to the intricate relationship between mental processes and physical health. This connection emphasizes how our thoughts, emotions, and beliefs can significantly influence physical well-being. Research has shown that stress, anxiety, and negative thoughts can lead to various health issues, including heart disease, obesity, and weakened immune function. Conversely, positive mental states, such as optimism and resilience, can enhance our overall health, increase longevity, and improve our quality of life.

Understanding the mind-body connection involves acknowledging how psychological factors impact physiological responses. For instance, when faced with stress, the body enters a fight-or-flight mode, releasing hormones such as cortisol and adrenaline. While these responses are beneficial in short bursts, chronic stress can lead to detrimental effects on health. Learning to manage stress through techniques such as mindfulness, meditation, and deep-breathing exercises can help restore balance and promote a healthier mind-body dynamic.

Moreover, the role of physical activity in strengthening the mind-body connection cannot be overlooked. Exercise has been proven to release endorphins, which are natural mood lifters, reducing feelings of depression and anxiety. Regular physical activity also enhances cognitive function, improves sleep patterns, and fosters social connections, all of which contribute to better mental health. By incorporating regular exercise into daily routines, individuals can cultivate a stronger and more resilient mind-body relationship.

Nutrition also plays a crucial role in the mind-body connection. The foods we consume can influence our mood and cognitive function. Diets rich in whole grains, fruits, vegetables, and healthy fats are associated with improved mental health outcomes. For example, omega-3 fatty acids found in fish have been linked to lower rates of depression and anxiety. Being mindful of dietary choices can empower individuals to foster a better mind-body connection, leading to enhanced well-being and longevity.

Finally, nurturing the mind-body connection requires a holistic approach integrating mental, emotional, and physical health practices. Engaging in activities that promote relaxation, such as yoga, tai chi, or creative arts, can help individuals connect more deeply with their bodies and minds. Additionally, fostering healthy relationships and seeking social support can provide emotional resilience. By embracing the mind-body connection, individuals can take proactive steps toward living longer and better, achieving a balanced and fulfilling life.

## Stress Management Techniques

Stress management is crucial for maintaining overall health and well-being, especially for those aiming to live longer and better lives. Stress has a significant impact on physical and mental health, leading to issues such as high blood pressure, anxiety, and weakened immune responses. Understanding and implementing effective stress management techniques can help individuals navigate life's challenges more effectively, thereby enhancing their quality of life and longevity.

One of the most effective techniques for managing stress is mindfulness meditation. This practice encourages individuals to focus on the present moment, fostering a sense of calm and reducing anxiety. Individuals can cultivate a greater awareness of their thoughts and emotions by dedicating just a few minutes each day to mindfulness exercises, such as deep breathing or guided imagery. This practice helps reduce stress and promotes emotional resilience, enabling individuals to handle difficult situations with a clearer mind and a more balanced perspective.

Physical activity is another powerful tool for stress management. Regular exercise releases endorphins, the body's natural mood lifters, which can create feelings of happiness and euphoria. Whether it's a brisk walk, yoga, or a more vigorous workout, engaging in physical activity helps to alleviate tension and improve overall mental health. Additionally, exercise can serve as a productive distraction, allowing individuals to take a break from stressors and focus on their physical well-being, which is essential for a long and healthy life.

Social support plays a vital role in managing stress effectively. Building and maintaining strong relationships with friends, family, and community can provide a safety net during challenging times. Engaging in conversations, sharing experiences, and seeking advice from loved ones can help individuals gain new perspectives on their stressors. Joining support groups or community organizations can further enhance this network, allowing individuals to connect with others who share similar challenges and experiences, fostering a sense of belonging and reducing feelings of isolation.

Lastly, the incorporation of hobbies and leisure activities into daily routines can significantly reduce stress levels. Engaging in activities that bring joy and fulfillment, such as reading, gardening, or painting, allows individuals to express themselves creatively and take a break from their daily responsibilities. These enjoyable pursuits can serve as a valuable outlet for stress relief, providing opportunities for relaxation and mental rejuvenation. Individuals can create a balanced lifestyle that supports long-term health and well-being by prioritizing leisure and personal interests.

## The Role of Mindfulness and Meditation

In recent years, mindfulness and meditation have gained significant attention for their potential benefits in enhancing well-being and promoting longevity. At its core, mindfulness involves the practice of being fully present and engaged in the moment without judgment. This simple yet profound practice encourages individuals to observe their thoughts, feelings, and physical sensations, fostering a greater awareness of their internal and external environments. By cultivating mindfulness, individuals can develop a deeper connection with themselves, leading to improved emotional regulation, reduced stress levels, and a greater sense of peace.

Meditation, a practice closely linked to mindfulness, involves focused attention and the cultivation of a calm and clear mind. Various forms of meditation exist, including mindfulness meditation, loving-kindness meditation, and transcendental meditation, each offering unique approaches to fostering awareness and relaxation. Regular meditation practice has been shown to alter brain structure and function, enhancing areas associated with emotional regulation, self-awareness, and cognitive flexibility. These changes can contribute to better decision-making and resilience in the face of life's challenges, which are essential for maintaining a healthy and balanced life.

The physiological impacts of mindfulness and meditation are equally noteworthy. Research indicates that these practices can lead to reductions in chronic stress, which is known to be a significant contributor to various health issues, including cardiovascular disease, obesity, and autoimmune disorders. Lowering cortisol levels and promoting relaxation, mindfulness, and meditation can enhance immune function and promote better overall health. These practices also encourage healthier lifestyle choices, such as improved diet and increased physical activity, further supporting the pursuit of longevity.

Incorporating mindfulness and meditation into daily routines does not require extensive time commitments or special training. Simple practices, such as mindful breathing or short guided meditations, can be easily integrated into everyday life. Even just a few minutes of focused attention on the breath can provide immediate stress relief and clarity. Moreover, many resources are available, including apps, online courses, and local classes, making these practices accessible to everyone, regardless of their background or experience level.

Ultimately, embracing mindfulness and meditation can serve as powerful tools for those seeking to enhance their quality of life and longevity. By fostering a greater sense of awareness, reducing stress, and promoting healthier lifestyle choices, these practices can lead to profound changes in both mental and physical health. As individuals learn to navigate the complexities of life with greater ease, they may find themselves living longer and living better, fully engaging in the richness of each moment.

## The Power of Your Subconscious Mind

The subconscious mind is a powerful entity that plays a significant role in our daily lives, influencing thoughts, behaviors, and overall well-being. It operates beneath our conscious awareness, storing beliefs, memories, and experiences that shape how we view the world. Understanding the power of your subconscious mind can be a crucial step towards achieving a longer, healthier life. By tapping into this reservoir of thoughts and emotions, individuals can foster positive changes that contribute to longevity and improved quality of life.

One of the primary functions of the subconscious mind is to process and store information. This includes both positive and negative experiences that can affect mental health and physical well-being. For instance, if someone has repeatedly experienced stress or trauma, these experiences may manifest as health issues later in life. Conversely, positive affirmations and experiences can lead to better health outcomes. Individuals can reprogram their mental frameworks by consciously feeding the subconscious with constructive thoughts and affirmations, leading to healthier choices and behaviors.

The subconscious also plays a vital role in motivation and habit formation. Many of our daily habits are driven by subconscious patterns established over time. For example, people who view exercise as an integral part of their lives are likelier to consistently engage in physical activity. By cultivating a positive mindset and embedding healthy habits into the subconscious, individuals can create a lifestyle conducive to longevity. This may involve visualization techniques, where one imagines engaging in healthy activities, reinforcing the desire to make those activities a reality.

Stress management is another critical aspect influenced by the subconscious mind. Chronic stress can lead to various health issues, including cardiovascular disease and weakened immune function. Learning to access and calm the subconscious can significantly reduce stress levels. Techniques such as meditation, mindfulness, and deep-breathing exercises help individuals tap into their subconscious, promoting relaxation and mental clarity. By addressing stress at its root, individuals can improve their overall well-being and increase their chances of living longer.

Ultimately, harnessing the power of the subconscious mind requires consistent effort and practice. Engaging in activities that promote self-awareness, such as journaling and reflective thinking, can help individuals understand their subconscious patterns. Additionally, seeking professional guidance through therapy or coaching can provide tools to unlock this potential. By recognizing and utilizing the power of the subconscious, individuals can create a positive feedback loop that enhances their physical, mental, and emotional health, paving the way for a longer, more fulfilling life.

## Using Your Conscious Mind to Program Your Subconscious Mind to Live Long

The conscious mind plays a pivotal role in shaping our beliefs, attitudes, and behaviors, all of which can significantly influence our lifespan and overall quality of life. By actively engaging with our conscious thoughts, we can program our subconscious mind to adopt healthier habits and a positive outlook on aging. This process begins with understanding the power of intention and how our daily choices can either support or undermine our long-term wellness. Deliberately focusing on positive affirmations and visualizations can create a mental framework that promotes longevity.

Visualization is a powerful tool for programming the subconscious mind. When we envision ourselves living a long and fulfilling life, we send a clear message to our subconscious about our desires and goals. This exercise can involve imagining ourselves engaging in activities that promote health, such as exercising, eating nutritious foods, and participating in social interactions. As these vivid images become ingrained in our subconscious, they begin to influence our behaviors and decision-making processes, making it easier to adopt a lifestyle conducive to longevity.

Affirmations are another effective method for reprogramming the subconscious. By regularly repeating positive statements about health and longevity, we can challenge and replace any limiting beliefs that may hinder our progress. For instance, affirmations such as "I am strong and healthy" or "Every day, I make choices that support my well-being" can reinforce a mindset focused on vitality. Over time, these affirmations can shift our subconscious beliefs, encouraging us to make choices that align with a longer, healthier life.

Mindfulness practices, such as meditation and deep breathing, also play a crucial role in programming the subconscious mind. These techniques help us cultivate awareness of our thoughts and emotions, allowing us to identify and release negative patterns that may be detrimental to our health. By fostering a state of calm and clarity, we can better align our conscious intentions with our subconscious programming. This alignment is essential for creating a lifestyle that prioritizes longevity and well-being.

Finally, consistency is key in this journey of reprogramming the subconscious mind. It is important to integrate these practices into our daily routines to reinforce positive changes. Whether through visualization, affirmations, or mindfulness, establishing a regular practice can solidify the connection between our conscious desires and subconscious beliefs. As we commit to this process, we gradually cultivate a mindset that embraces longevity, ultimately leading to a richer, healthier life.

# Chapter 5
# Social Connections and Longevity

**Building Strong Relationships**

Building strong relationships is a fundamental aspect of living a longer and healthier life. Research consistently shows that social connections significantly contribute to overall well-being and longevity. Individuals with robust social ties tend to experience lower levels of stress, improved mental health, and greater happiness.

This is because relationships provide emotional support, a sense of belonging, and opportunities for shared experiences, all of which are essential for maintaining a positive outlook on life.

One of the key elements in building strong relationships is effective communication. Open and honest dialogue fosters trust and understanding between individuals. It is essential to actively listen to others and express thoughts and feelings clearly. Engaging in meaningful conversations allows for deeper connections and helps to resolve potential conflicts before they escalate. Moreover, non-verbal communication plays a crucial role; body language, facial expressions, and eye contact can all enhance the quality of interactions and reinforce the messages being conveyed.

Another important aspect of nurturing relationships is investing time and effort into them. Regularly reaching out to friends and family, whether through phone calls, texts, or in-person visits, demonstrates that you value the relationship. Shared activities, such as dining together, participating in hobbies, or simply enjoying nature, can create lasting memories and strengthen bonds. It is also vital to be present during these interactions, putting away distractions to engage fully with one another and show genuine interest in each other's lives.

Furthermore, cultivating empathy and understanding can greatly enhance relationships. Recognizing and validating the feelings of others fosters a supportive environment where individuals feel safe to express themselves. Practicing kindness and patience, especially during challenging times, can solidify connections and build resilience within relationships. It is important to remember that everyone experiences ups and downs, and being there for one another can make a significant difference.

In conclusion, strong relationships are pivotal for a long and fulfilling life. By prioritizing effective communication, investing time, and practicing empathy, individuals can cultivate connections that enrich their lives. As we navigate through life, these relationships not only provide support but also enhance our overall quality of life, contributing to a sense of purpose and belonging that is vital for longevity and happiness.

## Community Engagement

Community engagement plays a vital role in enhancing the quality of life for individuals, particularly as they age. It encompasses participation in various social, cultural, and civic activities that foster connections among people. This engagement can take many forms, including volunteering, attending community events, and joining local clubs or organizations. When individuals actively participate in their communities, they often experience increased feelings of belonging and purpose, essential components of a fulfilling life.

Research shows that social connections can significantly impact longevity. Engaging with others helps to reduce feelings of isolation and depression, common challenges faced by older adults. By participating in community activities, individuals build relationships and provide and receive support. This reciprocal exchange enhances mental well-being and encourages a sense of responsibility towards one another, creating a supportive environment that can contribute to a longer, healthier life.

Active community involvement can also lead to improved physical health. Many community programs focus on physical activity, such as walking groups, fitness classes, or gardening clubs. These initiatives encourage participants to stay active, which is crucial for maintaining mobility and overall health as one grows older. Furthermore, being part of a group can motivate individuals to commit to their health goals, making exercise a more enjoyable and social experience.

In addition to the personal benefits, community engagement has broader implications for societal well-being. When individuals come together to support local causes, they strengthen the fabric of their neighborhoods. This collective effort can lead to improvements in local resources, such as parks, libraries, and healthcare services. Communities prioritizing engagement tend to be more resilient, with residents who care about each other and work collaboratively to address challenges. This sense of community can create a more vibrant and supportive environment for all residents, ultimately enhancing the quality of life for everyone.

To foster community engagement, it is essential for individuals to seek out opportunities that resonate with their interests and values. Local organizations, clubs, and volunteer programs often welcome new participants. Additionally, individuals can initiate their own community projects, bringing like-minded people together to address specific needs or interests. By taking the first step towards engagement, individuals enrich their lives and contribute to a culture that prioritizes connection, support, and longevity for all.

## The Impact of Loneliness

Loneliness is increasingly recognized as a significant public health issue that affects individuals across all age groups. Research has shown that loneliness can lead to a range of negative health outcomes, including increased risk of cardiovascular disease, weakened immune function, and even premature death. The psychological effects of loneliness are equally concerning, often leading to depression, anxiety, and a decline in cognitive function. Understanding the impact of loneliness is essential for promoting healthier, longer lives.

One of the primary ways loneliness affects health is through its influence on stress levels. When individuals experience loneliness, their bodies can respond with heightened stress responses, which include the release of cortisol, a hormone that, in excess, can damage various bodily systems. This chronic stress may contribute to inflammation, a factor linked to numerous health conditions such as arthritis, diabetes, and heart disease. Therefore, addressing loneliness is not just about improving social connections; it is also crucial for mitigating the physiological stressors that can undermine overall health.

Social isolation, a close relative to loneliness, has similarly dire consequences. Individuals who lack meaningful social interactions are more likely to experience a decline in mental health and physical well-being. Studies have indicated that social isolation can be as harmful to health as smoking 15 cigarettes a day. For older adults, the risks are particularly pronounced, as isolation can lead to a decline in mobility, increased risk of falls, and a greater likelihood of developing dementia. Maintaining social connections is vital for maintaining mental and physical health, especially as we age.

Moreover, the impact of loneliness extends beyond individual health; it can affect entire communities. When people feel isolated, they may disengage from community activities, which diminishes social cohesion and support networks. This disengagement can lead to a cycle where loneliness becomes normalized, making it more challenging for individuals to seek help or form new relationships. Encouraging community engagement and creating environments that foster connections can combat this trend, ultimately leading to healthier populations.

To effectively address loneliness, proactive measures are necessary. Interventions can range from community programs aimed at increasing social interaction to individual strategies like volunteering or joining clubs. Mental health resources should also be readily accessible to help individuals cope with feelings of loneliness and develop better social skills. By recognizing the profound impact of loneliness and taking steps to mitigate it, individuals and communities can enhance overall well-being and contribute to a longer, healthier life.

# Chapter 6
# Sleep and Recovery

**The Importance of Sleep**

Sleep is a fundamental biological necessity that plays a crucial role in overall health and well-being. During sleep, the body undergoes vital processes such as tissue repair, muscle growth, and protein synthesis. These functions are essential not only for physical health but also for maintaining cognitive function and emotional stability. Lack of adequate sleep can lead to a range of health issues, including obesity, diabetes, cardiovascular diseases, and weakened immune responses, all of which can significantly impact longevity.

The relationship between sleep and mental health is equally significant. Quality sleep contributes to improved mood regulation and cognitive performance. During sleep, the brain processes information from the day, consolidating memories and helping in problem-solving. Insufficient sleep can exacerbate stress, anxiety, and depression, leading to a cycle that adversely affects both mental and physical health. Prioritizing restorative sleep is, therefore, vital for maintaining emotional resilience and mental clarity throughout life.

Moreover, sleep is intricately linked to metabolic health. Research has shown that insufficient sleep can disrupt hormonal balance, particularly hormones that regulate appetite and metabolism, such as ghrelin and leptin. This disruption can lead to increased cravings for unhealthy foods, weight gain, and an elevated risk of metabolic syndrome. Understanding the importance of sleep in regulating these processes can encourage individuals to adopt healthier sleep habits, ultimately contributing to a longer, healthier life.

In addition to the physiological benefits, sleep also enhances productivity and performance in daily activities. Well-rested individuals are generally more focused, creative, and efficient. They can respond better to challenges and make more informed decisions. This increased productivity enhances personal satisfaction and achievement and can have a positive ripple effect on professional and social interactions, fostering a more fulfilling lifestyle overall.

In conclusion, recognizing the importance of sleep is essential for anyone seeking to live longer and better. Individuals can take proactive steps toward improving their health and quality of life by prioritizing sleep and understanding its multifaceted benefits. Establishing consistent sleep patterns, creating a restful environment, and practicing relaxation techniques can all contribute to better sleep hygiene. Embracing these practices can lead to enhanced physical health, improved mental well-being, and a greater capacity for resilience, ultimately paving the way for a longer, more fulfilling life.

## Sleep Hygiene Practices

Sleep hygiene practices are essential for maintaining the quality of sleep and overall health and well-being. Good sleep hygiene encompasses a variety of habits and environmental factors that can significantly affect how well you sleep. By adopting these practices, individuals can improve their sleep duration and quality, which are crucial components of a healthy lifestyle. These practices are especially important for those looking to live longer, as poor sleep is linked to several chronic conditions.

One of the foundational aspects of sleep hygiene is establishing a consistent sleep schedule. This means going to bed and waking up at the same time every day, even on weekends. Consistency helps regulate the body's internal clock, making it easier to fall asleep and wake up naturally. Creating a pre-sleep routine can also signal the body that it is time to wind down. Activities such as reading, taking a warm bath, or practicing relaxation techniques can help prepare the mind and body for restful sleep.

The sleep environment plays a crucial role in sleep hygiene. A comfortable, quiet, and dark room can significantly enhance sleep quality. Investing in a good mattress and pillows that provide adequate support is advisable. Keeping the bedroom cool can also promote better sleep, as cooler temperatures have been shown to facilitate the body's natural sleeping processes. Additionally, reducing exposure to screens and bright lights in the hour leading up to bedtime can help the body produce melatonin, the hormone responsible for regulating sleep.

Mindful consumption of food and beverages can further improve sleep hygiene. It is recommended to avoid large meals, caffeine, and alcohol close to bedtime. Caffeine, found in coffee, tea, and some sodas, can disrupt sleep patterns, while alcohol may initially make one feel sleepy but can lead to disrupted sleep later in the night. Instead, consider light snacks that promote sleep, such as those rich in magnesium or tryptophan, which can help the body relax and prepare for sleep.

Lastly, managing stress and anxiety through various relaxation techniques can greatly enhance sleep hygiene. Practices such as mindfulness meditation, deep breathing exercises, or gentle yoga can reduce stress levels and promote a sense of calm. Incorporating these practices into your daily routine improves sleep quality and contributes to overall mental and emotional health. By prioritizing sleep hygiene, individuals can take proactive steps toward a longer, healthier life, ensuring they are rested and ready to engage fully in their daily activities.

## Recovery Techniques for Optimal Health

Recovery techniques play a crucial role in achieving optimal health and longevity. As people age, the body's ability to recover from physical or mental stressors becomes increasingly important. Incorporating effective recovery strategies can enhance overall well-being, improve resilience, and reduce the risk of chronic diseases. This subchapter explores various recovery techniques that can be easily integrated into daily life, benefiting individuals of all ages and lifestyles.

One of the most fundamental recovery techniques is adequate sleep. Quality sleep is vital for physical and mental restoration. During sleep, the body undergoes critical processes such as tissue repair, muscle growth, and the consolidation of memories. Establishing a consistent sleep schedule, creating a relaxing bedtime routine, and ensuring a comfortable sleep environment can significantly enhance sleep quality. Additionally, limiting exposure to screens before bedtime and reducing caffeine intake can help individuals achieve deeper and more restorative sleep, ultimately contributing to better health and longevity.

Another essential recovery technique is proper nutrition. The foods we consume significantly affect our body's recovery processes. A balanced diet rich in whole foods, including fruits, vegetables, lean proteins, and healthy fats, provides the necessary nutrients that support recovery. Antioxidant-rich foods, such as berries and leafy greens, can help combat oxidative stress, while omega-3 fatty acids found in fish and nuts promote inflammation reduction. Staying hydrated is equally important, as water aids in digestion and nutrient absorption. Individuals can enhance their recovery and overall health by prioritizing nutrition.

Physical activity is also a vital component of recovery. Regular exercise not only strengthens the body but also promotes recovery through improved circulation and muscle repair. Activities such as yoga and stretching can enhance flexibility and reduce tension, while moderate aerobic exercise stimulates the release of endorphins, which can elevate mood and reduce stress. Incorporating rest days and active recovery sessions into an exercise routine allows the body to repair and rejuvenate, ensuring that individuals remain energized and healthy over the long term.

Mindfulness and stress management techniques are essential for facilitating mental and emotional recovery. Practices such as meditation, deep breathing exercises, and progressive muscle relaxation can help individuals manage stress levels effectively. These techniques promote a state of calmness and awareness, allowing the body to recover from the mental strains of daily life. Additionally, engaging in hobbies or spending time in nature can provide a much-needed break from routine stressors, further enhancing recovery. By incorporating mindfulness practices into daily life, individuals can foster a greater sense of well-being and improve their overall health.

# Chapter 7
## Preventive Healthcare

**Regular Check-Ups and Screenings**

Regular check-ups and screenings play a crucial role in maintaining health and enhancing longevity. These proactive measures enable individuals to detect potential health issues before they escalate into more serious conditions. By engaging in routine medical visits, people can work collaboratively with healthcare providers to monitor their health status, discuss any concerns, and adjust lifestyle choices as needed. The importance of these appointments cannot be overstated, as they serve as a foundation for a healthier life, allowing for early intervention and improved outcomes.

One of the key components of regular check-ups is the comprehensive evaluation of vital health metrics. Healthcare professionals assess blood pressure, cholesterol levels, body mass index, and other vital signs during these visits. This data provides a snapshot of overall health and helps identify risk factors for chronic diseases such as diabetes, heart disease, and hypertension. By understanding these risks, individuals can make informed decisions about their health and adopt preventive measures that can significantly reduce the likelihood of developing serious conditions.

Screenings are essential in the early detection of various diseases, including cancer, diabetes, and cardiovascular issues. Depending on age, gender, and family history, specific screenings may be recommended at different stages of life. For example, mammograms for breast cancer, colonoscopies for colorectal cancer, and blood tests for diabetes are just a few examples of preventive screenings that can save lives. Staying informed about recommended screening schedules and discussing them with healthcare providers ensures that individuals take charge of their health and address any potential issues early on.

In addition to physical health assessments, regular check-ups provide an opportunity to discuss mental health and emotional well-being. Mental health is a critical aspect of overall health and can significantly impact one's quality of life. During check-ups, individuals should feel empowered to talk about stress, anxiety, depression, or any other emotional challenges they may face. Healthcare providers can offer resources, referrals, or strategies to help manage these issues, contributing to a more holistic approach to health that encompasses physical and mental well-being.

Finally, adopting a mindset that values regular check-ups and screenings is essential for fostering a healthier lifestyle. By prioritizing these appointments, individuals demonstrate a commitment to their health and longevity. Establishing a routine that includes annual or biannual visits can instill a sense of accountability and motivate individuals to maintain healthy habits. As part of a broader approach to living longer and better, regular check-ups and screenings empower people to take control of their health, leading to improved well-being and a higher quality of life.

## Understanding Health Risks

Understanding health risks is essential to leading a long and fulfilling life. Numerous factors contribute to our overall health, including genetics, lifestyle choices, and environmental influences. By recognizing and addressing these risks, individuals can take proactive steps toward improving their health outcomes. This understanding allows us to make informed choices that can significantly impact our longevity and quality of life.

Genetic predisposition plays a crucial role in determining health risks. Certain conditions, such as heart disease, diabetes, and some cancers, can run in families. While we cannot change our genetic makeup, awareness of these hereditary factors can motivate individuals to adopt healthier habits and undergo regular screenings. For instance, individuals with a family history of heart disease may choose to prioritize cardiovascular health through diet and exercise, thereby mitigating their risk.

Lifestyle choices are perhaps the most significant contributors to health risks. Factors such as diet, physical activity, smoking, and alcohol consumption can either protect against or exacerbate health issues. A well-balanced diet rich in fruits, vegetables, whole grains, and lean proteins can reduce the risk of chronic diseases. Regular physical activity strengthens the heart, improves mental health, and aids in weight management. Conversely, harmful habits like smoking and excessive drinking are linked to numerous health problems, including respiratory diseases and liver damage. Understanding these lifestyle implications is vital for individuals striving for longevity.

Environmental factors also influence health risks, often in ways that are less obvious but equally important. Exposure to pollutants, chemicals, and unsafe living conditions can lead to chronic health issues. Urban areas often present higher risks due to air and noise pollution, while rural settings may expose individuals to different environmental hazards. Recognizing these risks can encourage individuals to advocate for healthier environments through community initiatives or personal lifestyle adjustments, such as living in less polluted areas.

Finally, understanding health risks involves recognizing the importance of preventive care. Regular check-ups, screenings, and vaccinations play a significant role in the early detection and management of potential health issues. Individuals can take charge of their health by engaging with healthcare providers and staying informed about recommended health practices. This proactive approach helps identify risks early and fosters a sense of empowerment, enabling individuals to live longer, healthier lives.

# Chapter 8
# Healthy Habits for Everyday Life

**The Power of Routine**

Establishing a routine is one of the most effective strategies for enhancing overall well-being and longevity. Routines create a sense of stability and predictability in daily life, helping individuals manage stress and improve mental health. By incorporating positive habits into a structured schedule, people can cultivate an environment that promotes physical activity, healthy eating, and quality sleep. This consistency fosters a mindset geared toward wellness, making it easier to adhere to lifestyle changes that contribute to a longer, healthier life.

Incorporating regular physical activity into a daily routine profoundly benefits the body and mind. Whether it involves walking, cycling, or engaging in strength training, exercise promotes cardiovascular health, strengthens muscles, and enhances flexibility. Moreover, it releases endorphins, which can elevate mood and reduce feelings of anxiety and depression. By setting aside specific times for exercise, individuals can ensure that they prioritize movement as an integral part of their daily lives, leading to sustained energy levels and improved overall health.

Nutrition is another crucial component of a routine that can significantly impact longevity. Planning meals and eating regularly can help individuals make healthier food choices. Routines that prioritize whole foods, such as fruits, vegetables, whole grains, and lean proteins, can lead to better nutritional intake. Meal prepping can also reduce the temptation to opt for quick, unhealthy options. By making eating habits part of a daily schedule, individuals can reinforce their commitment to a balanced diet, ultimately supporting their long-term health goals.

Sleep hygiene is an often-overlooked aspect of routine that plays a vital role in longevity. Establishing regular sleep patterns, including consistent bedtimes and wake-up times, can improve sleep quality and duration. Quality sleep is essential for cognitive function, emotional regulation, and physical recovery. A well-structured nighttime routine can signal the body that it is time to wind down, promoting relaxation and better sleep. Prioritizing rest within the daily routine can increase productivity and enhance overall well-being.

Finally, routines can serve as a foundation for social connections, which are essential for emotional health. Setting aside time for family, friends, or community activities can foster relationships that provide support and a sense of belonging. Engaging with others in regular social activities can reduce feelings of loneliness and isolation, which are linked to various health challenges. By making social interactions a regular part of life, individuals can build a robust support network contributing to their happiness and longevity. Embracing the power of routine can be a transformative step toward living not just longer but better.

## Setting Realistic Goals

Setting realistic goals is a fundamental step in enhancing the quality and longevity of life. Many people are motivated by the idea of self-improvement but often set goals that are either too ambitious or vague, leading to frustration and disappointment. To foster a sustainable approach to personal growth, it is essential to establish specific, measurable, achievable, relevant, and time-bound goals. This framework provides clarity and allows individuals to track progress, ensuring that the goals align with their broader aspirations for a longer, healthier life.

One effective strategy for setting realistic goals is to start with small, incremental changes. For instance, instead of aiming to run a marathon within a few weeks, an individual might begin with a goal of walking for thirty minutes three times a week. This gradual approach makes the goal more achievable and builds confidence and motivation as milestones are reached. As individuals experience small successes, they are more likely to stay committed to their long-term health and wellness objectives, thereby reinforcing positive habits that contribute to longevity.

Another important aspect of goal setting is ensuring that the goals are relevant to one's personal values and lifestyle. Goals that resonate with an individual's passions and interests are more likely to be pursued with enthusiasm. For example, someone who enjoys cooking might set a goal to prepare one new healthy recipe each week. Such a goal not only promotes nutritious eating habits but also enhances the enjoyment of daily life. By aligning goals with personal values, individuals can create a more meaningful journey towards better health and well-being.

Additionally, it is crucial to remain flexible and adaptable as circumstances change. Life is inherently unpredictable, and unforeseen challenges can arise that may disrupt even the best-laid plans. Setting realistic goals includes the understanding that adjustments may be necessary. For instance, if an individual faces a health setback, they might need to modify their fitness goals. Being open to change allows individuals to maintain their motivation and continue making progress, even when faced with obstacles.

Lastly, celebrating achievements, no matter how small, is an essential part of the goal-setting process. Recognizing progress helps to reinforce positive behaviors and creates a sense of accomplishment. This can be as simple as keeping a journal to document successes or sharing accomplishments with friends and family. Celebrating milestones enhances motivation and serves as a reminder of the journey toward living a longer, healthier life. Individuals can cultivate resilience and commitment to their health and well-being by setting realistic goals and adopting a positive mindset.

## Overcoming Barriers to Healthy Living

Overcoming barriers to healthy living is essential for anyone aiming to improve their quality of life and longevity. Many individuals encounter obstacles that hinder their ability to adopt healthier habits, such as lack of time, financial constraints, limited access to resources, and misinformation about health practices. Recognizing these barriers is the first step in addressing them effectively. By understanding the common challenges, individuals can develop strategies to navigate these hurdles and create a sustainable path toward better health.

One significant barrier is the misconception that healthy living requires a complete overhaul of one's lifestyle. Many people believe they must make drastic changes to their diet and exercise routine to see benefits. This belief can lead to frustration and discouragement when immediate results are not evident. Instead, focusing on small, incremental changes that are easier to implement and maintain is crucial. Simple adjustments, such as incorporating more fruits and vegetables into meals, taking short walks, or practicing mindfulness, can significantly improve health over time.

Access to resources is another barrier that can affect healthy living. In some communities, fresh produce and healthy food options may be scarce, while others may lack safe spaces for physical activity. To overcome this, individuals can seek out community programs, farmers' markets, or local initiatives that promote health and well-being. Additionally, utilizing technology, such as fitness apps or online cooking classes, can provide valuable resources and support, making it easier to adopt a healthier lifestyle regardless of one's circumstances.

Financial constraints often play a significant role in the ability to live healthily. Many perceive healthy food options and fitness programs as expensive, which can deter individuals from making positive changes. However, numerous budget-friendly strategies can promote health without breaking the bank. Planning meals, buying in bulk, and choosing seasonal produce can make healthy eating more affordable. Moreover, engaging in free or low-cost physical activities, such as walking, jogging, or online workout videos, can provide effective alternatives to costly gym memberships or fitness classes.

Finally, the influence of social and cultural factors can present barriers to healthy living. Family habits, peer pressure, and cultural norms can shape one's attitudes toward health and wellness. To overcome these challenges, individuals can seek social support by connecting with like-minded peers or joining groups focused on health and wellness.

By fostering a supportive environment, individuals can encourage one another to make healthier choices and share resources, creating a community that values and prioritizes long-term health. Embracing these strategies helps overcome barriers and fosters a more profound commitment to living longer and living better.

# Chapter 9
# Embracing Change and Adaptability

**The Role of Resilience**

Resilience plays a crucial role in the pursuit of a long and fulfilling life. It is the capacity to recover quickly from difficulties and adapt to challenging circumstances. In the context of longevity, resilience influences how individuals respond to stressors and affect their physical health, mental well-being, and overall quality of life. Understanding the mechanisms of resilience can empower individuals to cultivate this trait, leading to better outcomes as they age.

Psychological resilience is often characterized by a positive mindset, emotional regulation, and the ability to navigate adversity. Those who demonstrate resilience tend to view challenges as opportunities for growth rather than insurmountable obstacles. Research indicates that resilient individuals are likelier to engage in healthy behaviors, maintain social connections, and seek support when needed. This proactive approach to life's challenges contributes to a stronger immune system, lower levels of chronic stress, and a reduced risk of age-related diseases.

Moreover, resilience can significantly impact mental health as individuals age. As people encounter various life transitions—such as retirement, the loss of loved ones, or health decline—resilient individuals are better equipped to cope with grief and change. They are more likely to find meaning and purpose in their experiences, fostering fulfillment and happiness. This psychological fortitude is essential for maintaining cognitive function and emotional stability, aspects that are vital for a high quality of life in later years.

The development of resilience is not solely an innate trait; it can be cultivated through intentional practices. Engaging in mindfulness and stress-reduction techniques can enhance one's ability to bounce back from adversity. Additionally, fostering strong social networks and community ties provides a support system that bolsters resilience. Encouraging lifelong learning and adaptability can also empower individuals to face new challenges with confidence, ultimately contributing to a more vibrant and healthier life as they age.

In conclusion, resilience is fundamental to living longer and better. It equips individuals with the tools to navigate life's inevitable challenges, promoting physical and mental health. By understanding and actively developing resilience, people can create a more robust foundation for a fulfilling life, regardless of the obstacles they may encounter. Embracing resilience enhances individual well-being and contributes to a more resilient society as a whole, where individuals support one another in their journeys toward longevity.

## Adapting to Life Transitions

Whether anticipated or unexpected, life transitions are an inevitable part of the human experience. From entering retirement to navigating the challenges of aging, each transition can significantly impact one's quality of life. Adapting to these changes is crucial for maintaining mental, emotional, and physical well-being. Recognizing the signs of transition and understanding the emotional responses that accompany them can help individuals prepare for the journey ahead.

One of the first steps in adapting to life transitions is acknowledging the change. This recognition can manifest as feelings of uncertainty, anxiety, or even excitement. It is essential to allow oneself to experience these emotions fully. Validating feelings is a healthy coping mechanism and a stepping stone toward finding constructive ways to manage them. Journaling, discussing feelings with trusted friends or family, or seeking guidance from a professional can provide clarity and support.

Another important aspect of adapting is staying connected with others. Social connections play a critical role in emotional resilience during times of transition. Engaging with friends, family, or community groups can provide a sense of belonging and support. Participating in social activities, volunteering, or joining clubs related to personal interests can foster new relationships and strengthen existing ones. These connections can serve as a buffer against the stress of change, offering comfort and practical assistance.

Moreover, maintaining a healthy lifestyle contributes significantly to one's ability to adapt. Regular physical activity, a balanced diet, and adequate sleep are fundamental in promoting overall well-being. Exercise, in particular, has been shown to reduce stress and enhance mood, making it easier to cope with life's challenges. Mindfulness practices, such as meditation or yoga, can also help manage anxiety and foster a sense of peace, enabling individuals to approach transitions with a positive mindset.

Finally, embracing a proactive approach to change can lead to personal growth and fulfillment. Viewing transitions not merely as obstacles but as opportunities for learning and self-discovery can transform one's experience. Setting new goals, pursuing hobbies, or even exploring new career paths can invigorate life and create a sense of purpose. By adopting a flexible mindset and being open to new possibilities, individuals can confidently navigate life transitions, ultimately leading to a richer and more satisfying existence.

## Lifelong Learning

Lifelong learning is an essential aspect of living a fulfilling and extended life. It encompasses the continuous, voluntary, and self-motivated pursuit of knowledge for personal or professional development. Engaging in lifelong learning can significantly enhance cognitive function, promote emotional well-being, and create a sense of purpose. As individuals age, the importance of remaining intellectually active becomes even more pronounced, as it contributes to maintaining mental acuity and delaying cognitive decline.

One of the primary benefits of lifelong learning is its impact on brain health. Studies indicate that engaging in mentally stimulating activities—such as reading, solving puzzles, or learning new skills—can strengthen neural connections and even foster the growth of new brain cells. This neuroplasticity is vital for older adults, as it helps counteract the natural aging process, keeping the mind sharp and resilient. By committing to learning new things, individuals can cultivate a proactive approach to their mental fitness, which is crucial for a longer, healthier life.

Moreover, lifelong learning fosters social connections and engagement, which are critical components of well-being. Participating in classes, workshops, or community events often leads to meeting new people and forming meaningful relationships. These social interactions can combat feelings of isolation and loneliness, which are prevalent among older adults. Building a network of like-minded individuals encourages continuous learning and provides emotional support, enhancing the overall quality of life.

Incorporating lifelong learning into daily routines can be as simple as setting aside time for reading, enrolling in online courses, or attending local lectures. Technology has made it easier than ever to access educational resources, allowing individuals to learn at their own pace and on their own schedule. Whether through podcasts, virtual classes, or mobile apps, there are countless opportunities to expand knowledge and skills. This flexibility empowers individuals to tailor their learning experiences to their interests and goals, ensuring the journey remains enjoyable and fulfilling.

Ultimately, embracing a mindset of lifelong learning is a commitment to personal growth and self-improvement. It encourages resilience, adaptability, and curiosity—traits that are invaluable in navigating the challenges of aging. By prioritizing education and exploration throughout life, individuals can not only enhance their longevity but also enrich their experiences, making the journey of living longer synonymous with living better. The pursuit of knowledge is a lifelong endeavor that can lead to a more vibrant, engaged, and meaningful existence.

# Chapter 10
# Inspiring Stories of Longevity

**Interviews with Centenarians**

Interviews with centenarians provide invaluable insights into the factors contributing to a long and fulfilling life. These individuals, having celebrated their 100th birthdays and beyond, possess a wealth of experiences and wisdom that can guide us in our quest for longevity. Their stories often reveal common themes, such as strong social connections, a sense of purpose, and the importance of maintaining an active lifestyle. By understanding their unique perspectives, we can glean practical advice for enhancing our own lives and potentially extending our years.

One of the most striking aspects of centenarians' lives is the emphasis they place on relationships. Many of them attribute their longevity to the close bonds they have maintained with family and friends. These connections not only provide emotional support but also foster a sense of belonging and community. For instance, one centenarian recounted how regular gatherings with family and friends helped keep her spirits high and her mind engaged. This underscores the idea that nurturing relationships can play a crucial role in promoting overall well-being and longevity.

Another common thread among centenarians is the importance of staying active, both physically and mentally. Many of these individuals have engaged in regular physical activity, whether walking, gardening, or participating in community sports. They emphasize that movement is not just about exercise; it is about maintaining a routine that keeps the body and mind sharp. Additionally, many centenarians partake in hobbies stimulating their intellect, such as reading, puzzles, or learning new skills. This highlights the idea that an active lifestyle is vital for sustaining health as we age.

A sense of purpose often emerges as a key factor in the lives of those who reach advanced ages. Centenarians often find meaning in various aspects of their daily lives, whether through work, volunteering, or caring for loved ones. One centenarian shared how his passion for painting gave him a reason to get up each day and express his creativity. This sense of purpose provides motivation and contributes to emotional and mental resilience, helping individuals navigate the challenges of aging.

Finally, many centenarians advocate for a balanced approach to life, emphasizing moderation in all things. They often speak about the importance of a healthy diet but highlight the value of indulging in treats from time to time. This philosophy extends to other areas of life, such as work-life balance and stress management. By prioritizing balance, centenarians demonstrate that longevity is not just about the number of years lived but also about the quality of those years. Their stories serve as a reminder that by fostering relationships, staying active, finding purpose, and maintaining balance, we can all aspire to live longer, healthier lives.

## Lessons from Longevity Hotspots

Longevity hotspots, often called Blue Zones, are regions worldwide where people live significantly longer and healthier lives. These areas, such as Okinawa in Japan, Sardinia in Italy, and Nicoya in Costa Rica, provide valuable insights into the factors that contribute to prolonged life expectancy. Studies of these regions reveal a combination of lifestyle choices, social structures, and dietary habits that can serve as a blueprint for anyone looking to enhance their own lifespan and well-being.

One of the most striking lessons from these longevity hotspots is the importance of a plant-based diet. In many of these regions, most food is consumed from fruits, vegetables, whole grains, and legumes. This diet is rich in essential nutrients and low in processed foods and sugars. People in Blue Zones tend to eat in moderation, often following the principle of "Hara Hachi Bu," which encourages them to stop eating when they are about 80% full. This mindful approach to eating can help manage weight and reduce the risk of chronic diseases.

Another critical factor observed in these regions is the role of physical activity and natural movement in daily life. Residents of longevity hotspots often engage in regular, low-intensity physical activities such as walking, gardening, or manual labor. This contrasts with the high-intensity workouts commonly promoted in many modern fitness regimes. The natural integration of movement into daily routines fosters physical health and social interaction, which is another key aspect of longevity.

Social connections and community support are also prominent in the lifestyles of those living in Blue Zones. Strong relationships with family, friends, and neighbors contribute significantly to emotional well-being and resilience. People in these regions often prioritize time spent with loved ones and engage in communal activities, which helps reduce stress and foster a sense of belonging. This social fabric is vital, providing emotional support and encouraging healthy behaviors, creating an environment conducive to long life.

Lastly, maintaining a sense of purpose is a common thread among the inhabitants of longevity hotspots. Many individuals in these areas have a clear sense of why they wake up in the morning, whether through work, family, or community involvement. This sense of purpose has been linked to lower levels of stress and better overall health. Individuals can enhance their mental and emotional health by cultivating a personal mission or engaging in activities that bring joy and fulfillment, paving the way toward a longer and more vibrant life.

**Personal Journeys to a Healthier Life**

Personal journeys to a healthier life often begin with a moment of realization or a significant life event that prompts individuals to reassess their current habits and lifestyles. These pivotal moments can range from a health scare to the birth of a child or even the loss of a loved one. Such experiences serve as catalysts, encouraging people to seek out better health practices. Understanding the motivation behind these transformations can inspire others to embark on their own paths toward improved well-being.

The process of adopting healthier habits is unique for everyone and is often influenced by personal circumstances, cultural backgrounds, and available resources. For some, it may involve a complete overhaul of their daily routines, including diet and exercise. For others, it might mean making small, manageable changes over time. The key is to find an approach that resonates with the individual, allowing for sustainable changes rather than quick fixes. This flexibility is crucial, as the journey to health is not a one-size-fits-all experience.

Support systems play a vital role in personal journeys to a healthier life. Whether it's friends, family, or community groups, having a network of encouragement can make a significant difference. Many individuals report that sharing their goals with others holds them accountable and provides motivation and affirmation. Participating in group activities, such as fitness classes or cooking workshops, fosters a sense of belonging and can make the journey more enjoyable and less isolating.

Tracking progress is another essential component of personal health journeys. Many individuals find value in documenting their efforts, whether through journals, apps, or social media. This practice not only allows for reflection but also helps in recognizing achievements, both big and small. Celebrating milestones, even minor ones, reinforces positive behaviors and helps maintain momentum. Furthermore, being able to look back on one's journey can provide motivation during challenging times.

Ultimately, personal journeys to healthier lives are about embracing change and fostering resilience. Unique challenges and triumphs mark each individual's path, but the underlying theme remains the same: the pursuit of better health is a lifelong commitment. By sharing stories and strategies, we can create a culture that values well-being and supports one another in living longer and better lives. This collective effort can inspire a broader movement towards healthful living, benefiting not just individuals but communities as a whole.

# Chapter 11
# Creating Your Personal Longevity Plan

## Assessing Your Current Lifestyle

Assessing your current lifestyle is a critical first step in the journey toward living a longer and healthier life. This process involves taking a comprehensive look at various aspects of your daily routine, habits, and overall well-being. By understanding where you currently stand, you can identify areas that require change and improvement. This self-assessment allows for a clearer path toward adopting healthier practices and making informed decisions that can positively impact longevity.

Begin by evaluating your dietary habits. What you eat plays a significant role in your overall health and can either promote longevity or lead to health issues. Take note of your daily food intake, paying attention to the balance of nutrients, portion sizes, and frequency of meals. Are you consuming a variety of fruits and vegetables? How often do you indulge in processed foods or sugary snacks? Keeping a weekly food diary can provide valuable insights into your eating patterns, helping you recognize healthy choices and areas needing adjustment.

Next, consider your physical activity levels. Regular exercise is a cornerstone of a healthy lifestyle and contributes significantly to longevity. Assess how much time you dedicate to physical activity each week. Are you meeting the recommended guidelines of at least 150 minutes of moderate aerobic activity? Look for opportunities to increase your activity, whether through structured workouts, walking more, or incorporating movement into your daily tasks. Remember, even small changes can lead to significant health benefits over time.

Mental and emotional well-being is another crucial aspect of lifestyle assessment. Stress management, social connections, and mental stimulation are vital for a fulfilling life. Reflect on how you handle stress and whether you have healthy coping mechanisms in place. Consider your social interactions and support networks, as strong relationships can enhance both mental health and longevity. Engaging in hobbies, reading, or learning new skills can also promote cognitive health and emotional resilience.

Finally, review your sleep patterns. Quality sleep is essential for overall health and longevity. Assess how many hours of sleep you get on average and the quality of that sleep. Are you waking up feeling rested? Poor sleep can lead to a myriad of health issues, so it is important to prioritize good sleep hygiene. Creating a consistent sleep schedule, optimizing your sleep environment, and limiting screen time before bed are all strategies to improve this vital aspect of your lifestyle. By thoroughly assessing your current lifestyle, you can create a solid foundation for making meaningful changes that support a longer and healthier life.

## Setting Your Longevity Goals

Setting your longevity goals is an essential step in taking control of your health and well-being as you age. Longevity goals can encompass various aspects of life, including physical health, mental well-being, social connections, and lifestyle choices. By establishing clear, achievable goals, you create a roadmap that can guide your daily habits and decisions. This proactive approach empowers you to make informed choices that align with your desire for a longer, healthier life.

To begin setting longevity goals, it is important to assess your current health status and lifestyle. Consider factors such as your diet, exercise routine, sleep quality, and stress levels. Reflect on your family history and any genetic predispositions that may influence your health. This self-assessment allows you to identify areas for improvement and to prioritize your goals accordingly. For example, if you find that you are not engaging in regular physical activity, a goal might be to incorporate at least 30 minutes of exercise into your daily routine.

Once you have identified specific areas of focus, it is crucial to set SMART goals—specific, measurable, achievable, relevant, and time-bound. This framework helps ensure that your goals are realistic and attainable. For instance, instead of setting a vague goal like "eat healthier," you could aim to include three servings of fruits and vegetables in your daily diet for the next month. This specificity not only clarifies your intentions but also allows you to track your progress, making it easier to stay motivated.

In addition to physical health, consider setting goals that enhance your mental and emotional well-being. Practices such as mindfulness, meditation, and lifelong learning can significantly contribute to a fulfilling life. You might set a goal to read one book a month or to practice meditation for ten minutes each day. Engaging with your community and nurturing relationships can also be vital for longevity. Setting a goal to connect with friends or family members regularly can foster a support network that enriches your life and promotes emotional resilience.

Finally, revisit and adjust your longevity goals regularly. Life circumstances change, and what might have been a priority a year ago may no longer hold the same significance. By continuously evaluating your goals and making necessary adjustments, you ensure that they remain aligned with your evolving aspirations and lifestyle. Embracing this dynamic approach to goal setting not only enhances your chances of living a longer life but also contributes to a richer and more fulfilling experience as you navigate the journey of aging.

**Tracking Progress and Making Adjustments**

Tracking progress and making adjustments is a critical aspect of any long-term lifestyle change aimed at enhancing longevity and overall well-being. To achieve sustainable results, individuals must regularly assess their habits and outcomes. This process begins with identifying specific health goals, which can range from improving diet and increasing physical activity to enhancing mental health and managing stress. By establishing clear, measurable objectives, individuals create a roadmap that guides their journey toward a longer, healthier life.

One effective method for tracking progress is to maintain a health journal. This journal can include daily entries about nutrition, exercise routines, sleep patterns, and emotional well-being. By documenting these aspects, individuals can identify trends, recognize achievements, and pinpoint areas needing improvement. Additionally, digital tools and applications designed for health tracking can simplify this process. They often provide features that allow users to log their activities, set reminders, and visualize their progress through graphs and charts, making it easier to stay motivated.

Regularly reviewing the data collected in health journals or applications is essential for making informed adjustments to one's routine. This review process should occur weekly or monthly, depending on personal preferences and goals. During these reviews, individuals can evaluate what strategies have been effective and which may need alteration. For instance, if one finds that certain dietary changes lead to increased energy levels but struggles with consistency, it may be necessary to adapt meal planning or preparation methods to better fit lifestyle demands.

Flexibility is key when it comes to making adjustments. Life circumstances often change, and what works well today may not be suitable in the future. Therefore, being open to trying new approaches is vital. This might involve experimenting with different forms of exercise, exploring new healthy recipes, or incorporating mindfulness practices to enhance mental health. By embracing change and viewing setbacks as opportunities for growth, individuals can sustain their commitment to living longer and living better.

Ultimately, the process of tracking progress and making adjustments fosters a deeper understanding of one's body and mind. It encourages a proactive attitude toward health and reinforces the idea that longevity is not merely about the number of years lived but the quality of those years. By continuously assessing personal health journeys and making necessary adjustments, individuals can cultivate a fulfilling, vibrant life that aligns with their aspirations for longevity and well-being.

# Chapter 12:
# Conclusion: A Holistic Approach to Living Longer, Living Better

**Integrating All Aspects of Life**

Integrating all aspects of life is a crucial component in the pursuit of longevity and overall well-being. This holistic approach recognizes that various facets of life—physical health, mental wellness, social connections, and environmental factors—are interconnected and contribute to a person's quality of life. By understanding and nurturing these interrelationships, individuals can create a balanced lifestyle that not only promotes a longer life but enhances the quality of each day.

Physical health is often regarded as the foundation of longevity. Regular exercise, a balanced diet, and adequate sleep are essential for maintaining bodily functions and preventing chronic diseases. However, integrating physical health with mental wellness is equally important.

Practices such as mindfulness, meditation, and stress management techniques not only improve mental clarity but also enhance physical performance. When individuals prioritize both their physical and mental health, they are more likely to experience a sense of vitality that contributes to a longer life.

Social connections play a significant role in longevity. Humans are inherently social beings, and maintaining strong relationships can lead to increased happiness and reduced stress levels. Engaging with family, friends, and community fosters a support system that can provide emotional nourishment and practical help during challenging times. Furthermore, social interactions can stimulate cognitive function and promote a sense of belonging, both of which are integral to maintaining mental health as one ages. By integrating social activities into daily life, individuals can create a network that positively impacts their overall well-being.

Environmental factors also deserve attention in the conversation about longevity. The spaces in which we live and work can significantly affect our health. Access to green spaces, clean air, and safe neighborhoods contributes to physical activity and mental relaxation.

Additionally, establishing a home environment that promotes wellness—such as reducing clutter, enhancing natural light, and incorporating elements of nature—can create a sanctuary conducive to relaxation and rejuvenation. Integrating environmental consciousness into daily routines encourages a lifestyle that respects personal health and the planet, ultimately leading to a more fulfilling life.

Ultimately, integrating all aspects of life requires a commitment to self-awareness and continuous improvement. Individuals must regularly assess their physical health, mental wellness, social connections, and environmental influences to identify areas for growth. By adopting a proactive mindset and embracing change, people can create a comprehensive strategy that aligns with their values and goals. This holistic approach paves the way for a longer life and enriches the experiences that fill each day, leading to a life lived fully and vibrantly.

## The Future of Longevity Research

The future of longevity research is a rapidly evolving field that holds the promise of extending human lifespan while simultaneously enhancing the quality of life. As scientific advancements continue to accelerate, researchers are exploring various biological, genetic, and environmental factors that contribute to aging. These studies aim not only to understand the mechanisms of aging but also to identify interventions that can promote healthier aging and potentially delay the onset of age-related diseases. By integrating insights from diverse disciplines such as genetics, epidemiology, and biochemistry, the quest for longevity is becoming increasingly multifaceted.

One of the most significant areas of longevity research focuses on the role of genetics in aging. Scientists are uncovering specific genes that influence lifespan and health span, the period during which individuals remain healthy and free from serious illness. Studies on centenarians have revealed genetic variants that may confer resilience against age-related diseases. This knowledge can lead to the development of targeted therapies aimed at enhancing these protective factors, thus providing a potential pathway for extending life and improving health outcomes. As gene-editing technologies like CRISPR become more refined, the possibility of manipulating these genetic factors to promote longevity is becoming more tangible.

Another promising avenue is the study of cellular senescence, which refers to the process by which cells lose their ability to divide and function effectively. Accumulation of senescent cells in tissues is linked to inflammation and various age-related diseases. Researchers are investigating senolytics, compounds that selectively eliminate senescent cells, as a potential strategy to rejuvenate tissues and extend health span. Early clinical trials are already showing encouraging results, suggesting that targeting cellular senescence could be a key intervention in the quest for longevity. This approach emphasizes the importance of living longer and living better by reducing the burden of chronic diseases associated with aging.

Additionally, the impact of lifestyle factors on longevity continues to be a focus of research. Studies examining the effects of diet, exercise, and social connections illustrate that these factors significantly influence health outcomes as individuals age. The Mediterranean diet, for example, has been associated with a lower risk of heart disease and cognitive decline. Regular physical activity is linked to improved mental health and physical function in older adults. These findings underscore the importance of adopting healthy lifestyle habits as part of a comprehensive strategy for promoting longevity. As research continues to uncover the interplay between lifestyle and biological aging, practical recommendations can emerge to guide individuals toward healthier choices.

Lastly, technological advancements are poised to revolutionize longevity research and its applications. Artificial intelligence and machine learning are being harnessed to analyze vast datasets, identify patterns, and predict health outcomes based on genetic, environmental, and lifestyle factors. Wearable technology provides real-time data on health metrics, enabling personalized health interventions. Telemedicine and remote monitoring are making it easier for individuals to access healthcare tailored to their specific needs.

As these technologies become more integrated into everyday life, they can empower individuals to take charge of their health and well-being, potentially leading to longer, healthier lives. The future of longevity research is bright, promising not just an increase in lifespan but also an enhancement in the overall quality of life for all.

## A Call to Action for Healthier Living

The conversation around health and longevity has gathered momentum in recent years, highlighting the importance of making informed lifestyle choices that contribute to a longer and healthier life. A call to action for healthier living is essential for individual well-being and the collective health of our communities. By embracing a holistic approach to health, everyone can take meaningful steps toward enhancing their quality of life and longevity.

Physical activity plays a critical role in promoting longevity. Regular exercise, whether through structured workouts or everyday activities like walking, gardening, or dancing, can significantly improve cardiovascular health, boost mental well-being, and enhance overall vitality. The goal should be to incorporate at least 150 minutes of moderate-intensity aerobic activity per week, along with strength training exercises at least twice a week. For those new to exercise, starting with small, manageable goals can lead to sustainable habits that promote long-term health benefits.

Nutrition is another cornerstone of healthier living. A balanced diet rich in whole foods, including fruits, vegetables, whole grains, lean proteins, and healthy fats, is vital for maintaining energy levels and preventing chronic diseases. It is essential to limit the intake of processed foods, added sugars, and unhealthy fats. Educating oneself about nutritional choices and meal planning can empower individuals to make healthier decisions. By fostering an environment that encourages cooking at home and exploring diverse cuisines, communities can support each other in making better dietary choices.

Mental and emotional health are equally important in the quest for longevity. Stress management techniques, such as mindfulness, meditation, and deep-breathing exercises, can significantly impact one's overall health. Cultivating strong social connections and engaging in community activities can enhance emotional resilience and provide a support system. Recognizing the signs of mental health challenges and seeking help when needed is crucial. Individuals can create a balanced lifestyle that supports their physical health and longevity by prioritizing mental well-being.

Finally, preventive healthcare cannot be overlooked in the pursuit of a healthier life. Regular check-ups and screenings can detect potential health issues early, providing timely intervention. Staying informed about personal health metrics, such as blood pressure, cholesterol levels, and body mass index, empowers individuals to take control of their health. Encouraging everyone to prioritize preventive care can foster a culture of health awareness and proactive living, ultimately leading to a longer, more fulfilling life. The call to action is clear: adopt healthier habits today for a better tomorrow. It's a beautiful day.

Printed in Great Britain
by Amazon